Pretend You're a
Star

Karen Bryant-Mole

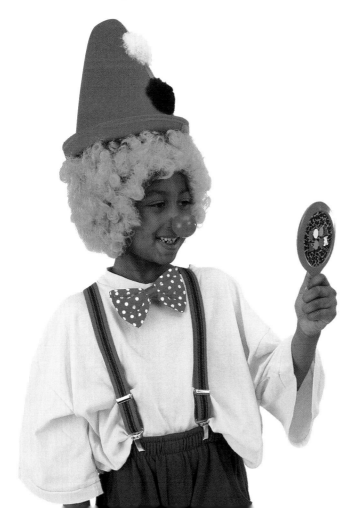

Heinemann Interactive Library
Des Plaines, Illinois

HE

Published by Heinemann Interactive Library,
an imprint of Reed Educational & Professional Publishing,
1350 East Touhy Avenue, Suite 240 West
Des Plaines, IL 60018

Produced by Times Offset (M) Sdn. Bhd.

Designed by Jean Wheeler

Commissioned photography by Zul Mukhida

02 01 00 99 98
10 9 8 7 6 5 4 3 2 1

Library of Congress Cataloging-in-Publication Data

Bryant-Mole, Karen.
    You're a star/Karen Bryant-Mole.
      p. cm. -- (Pretend)
    Includes biographical references and index.
    Summary: Explains what different kinds of performers do and
suggests ideas for pretending to be a magician, pop singer, acrobat,
juggler, clown, or other entertainer.
    ISBN 1-57572-186-4 (lib. bdg.)
    1. Performing arts--Juvenile literature. (1. Performing arts.)
I. Title. II. Series: Bryant-Mole, Karen. Pretend.
PN1584.B78 1997
791--dc21   97-20059
                                                                      CIP
                                                                       AC

Acknowledgments
The author and publishers are grateful to the following for permission to reproduce copyright photographs:
Cephas: 5 Stuart Boreham, 15 Nicholas James; Chapel Studios: 7 Timm Garrod, 11, 232 Graham Horner, 13 Tim Richardson; Eye Ubiquitous: 19 Mike Southern; Tony Stone Images: 9 Geoff Johnson, 21; Zefa: 17.

Cover photograph Zul Mukhida

Every effort has been made to contact copyright holders of any material reproduced in this book. Any omissions will be rectified in subsequent printings if notice is given to the publisher.

Words in bold, **like this**, are explained in the glossary on page 24.

Contents

13.95

Magician

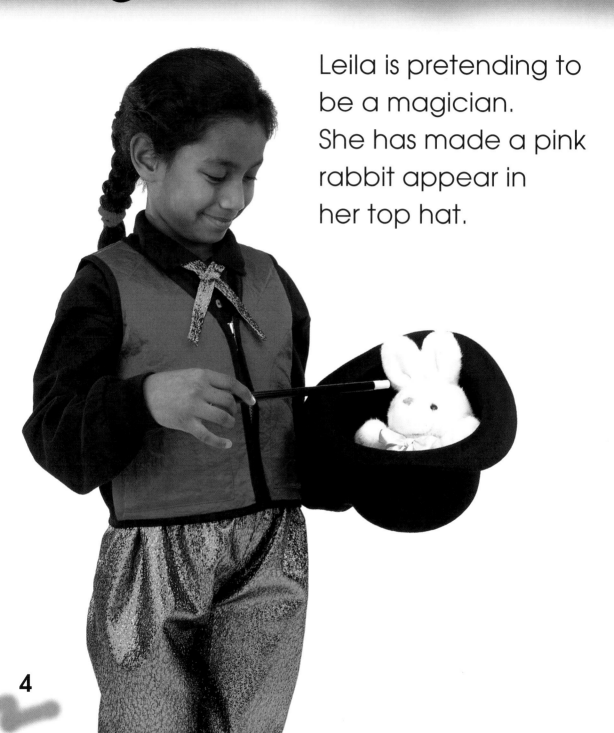

Leila is pretending to
be a magician.
She has made a pink
rabbit appear in
her top hat.

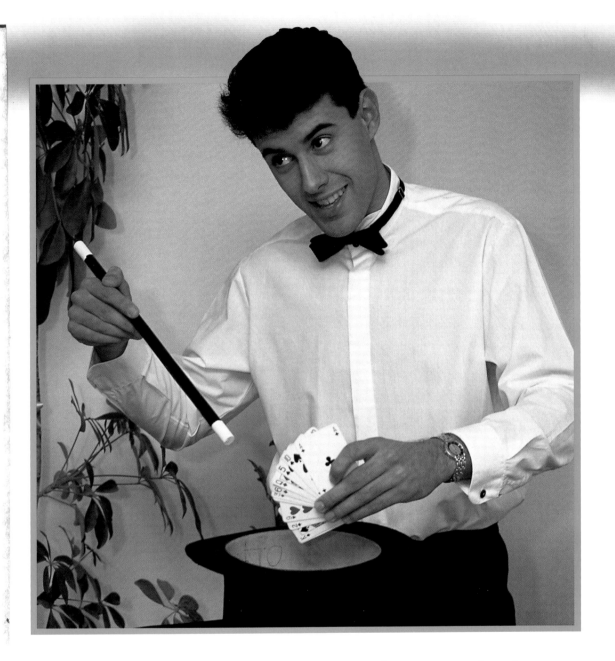

Magicians often use a magic wand when they make things appear and disappear. This magician can do card tricks, too.

Rock Singer

Ethan enjoys
pretending to be
a rock singer.
He is using a
hairbrush as his
microphone.

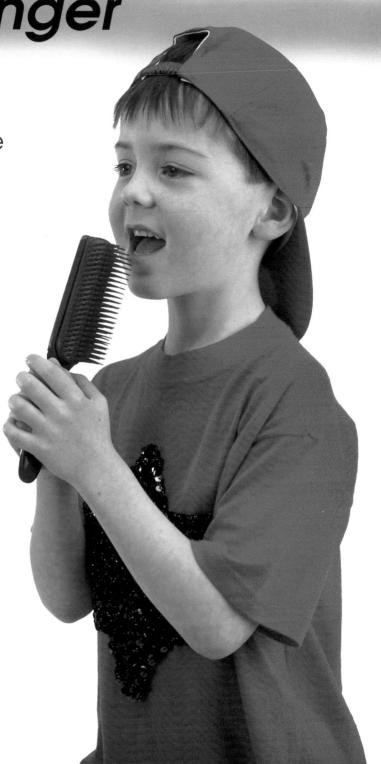

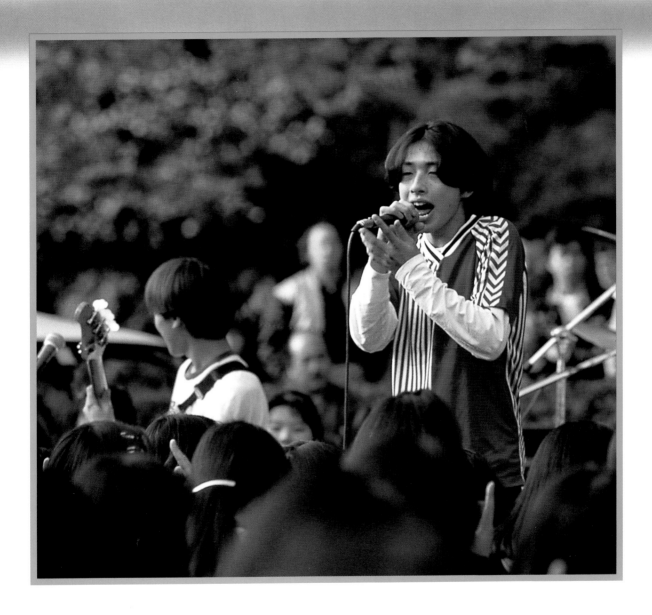

This singer is singing into a real microphone.
The microphone makes the singer's voice
sound louder.

Acrobat

Gemma is pretending to be an acrobat. She is trying to balance a plastic cup on her head!

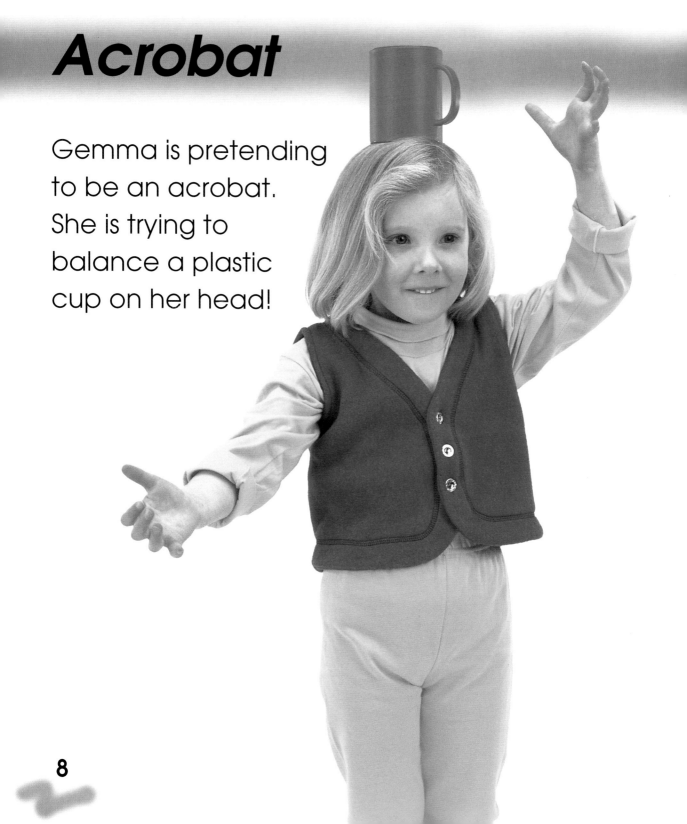

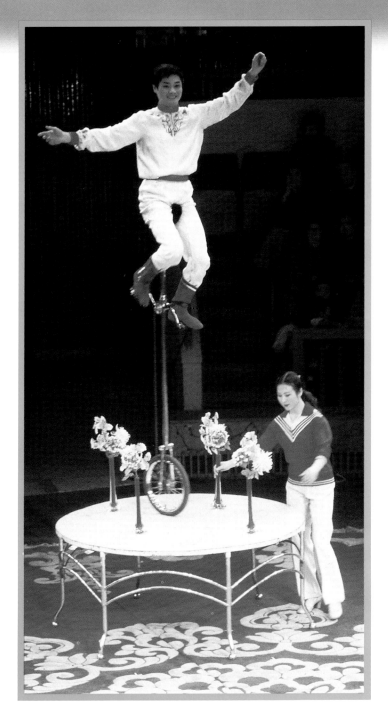

Acrobats have to be very good at balancing. This acrobat is balancing on a special cycle called a **unicycle**.

Band Player

Aliyu is marching
as he plays his
toy drum.
He is pretending
to be a band player.

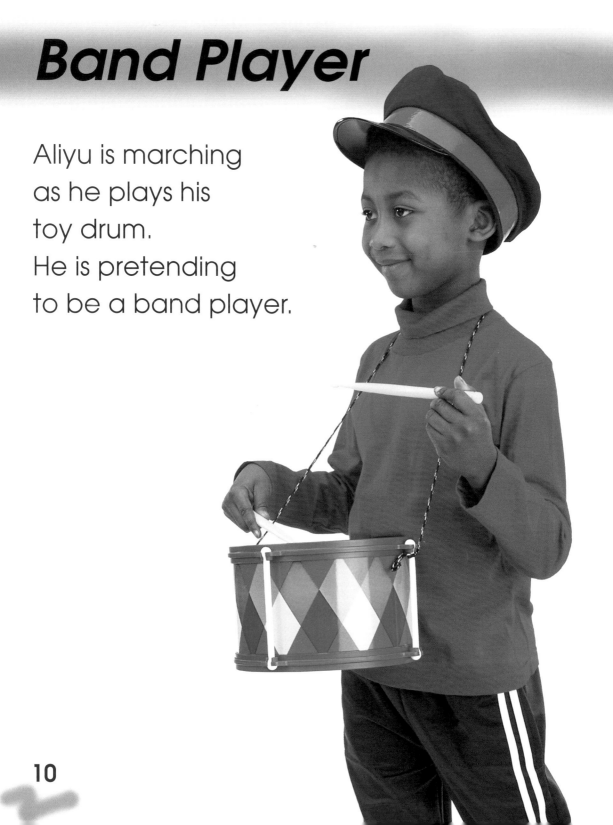

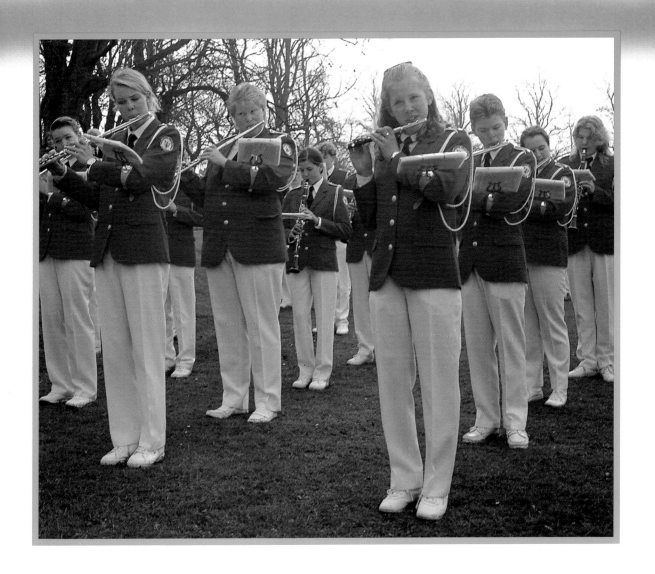

These band players can march, read the music, and play their **instruments**, all at the same time. They have their music in special holders on their sleeves.

Movie Star

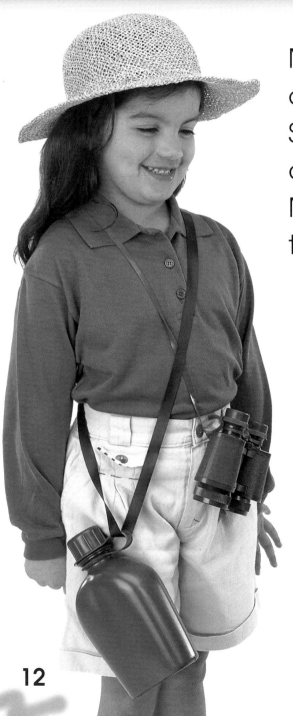

Melissa would like to be
a movie star.
She is dressed up like
an explorer.
Megan is pretending
to film her.

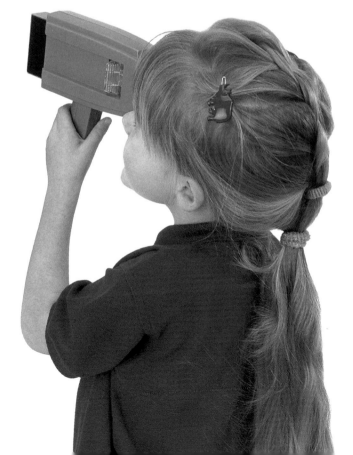

These actors are dressed
in **old-fashioned** clothes.
The man in front of the camera tells
everyone that the filming is about to start.

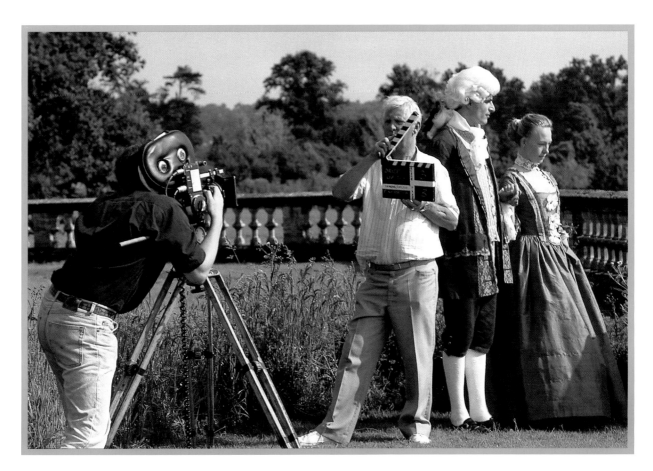

Puppeteer

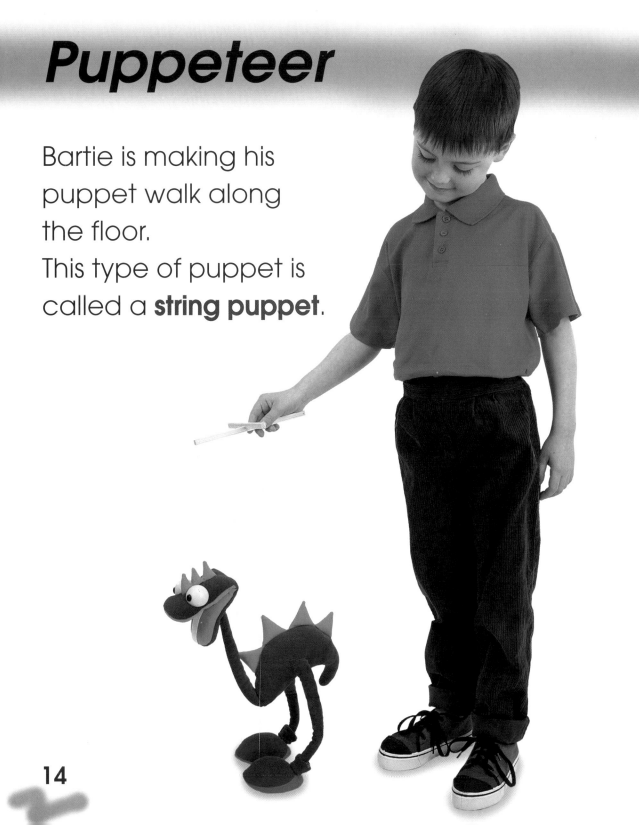

Bartie is making his puppet walk along the floor.
This type of puppet is called a **string puppet**.

14

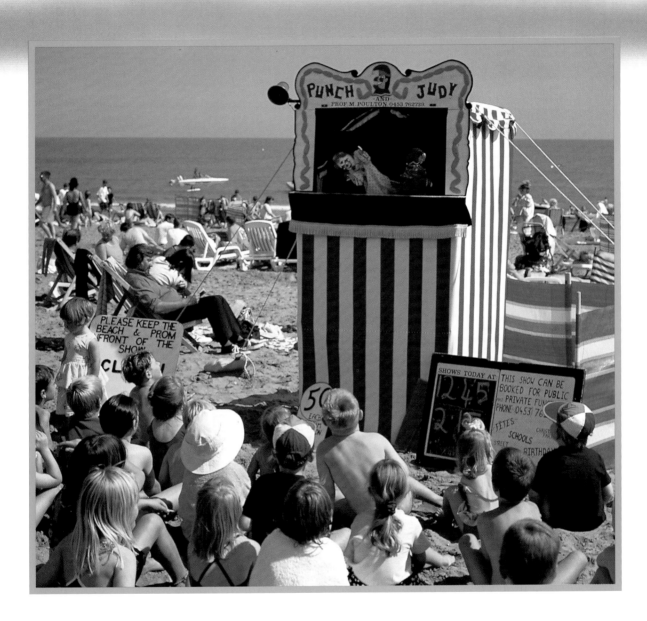

These puppets are called **glove puppets**. The person who is working the puppets is hidden inside the striped tent.

Ballet Dancer

Gemma wears a **tutu** when she pretends to be a ballet dancer. She is practicing pointing her toes.

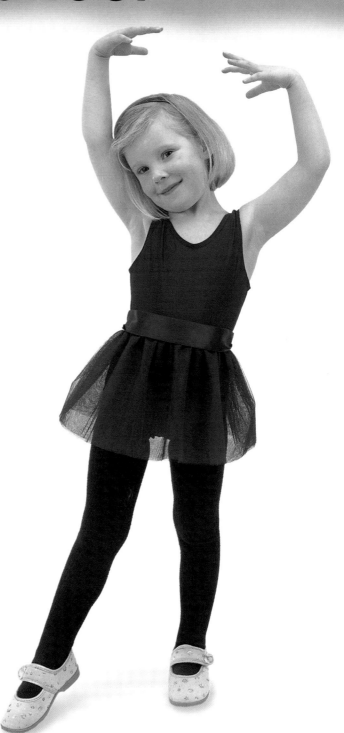

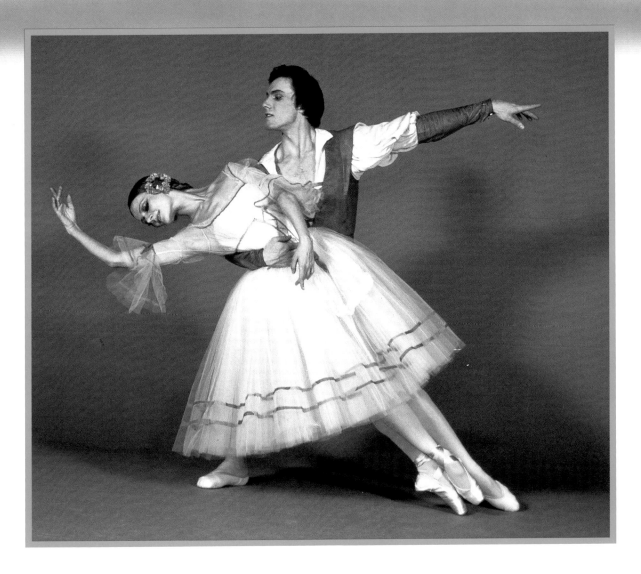

Real ballet dancers have to practice
for many hours every day.
It takes a lot of work to become as
good as these dancers.

Juggler

Leila is learning how to juggle.
She starts by learning how to
juggle with just two balls.

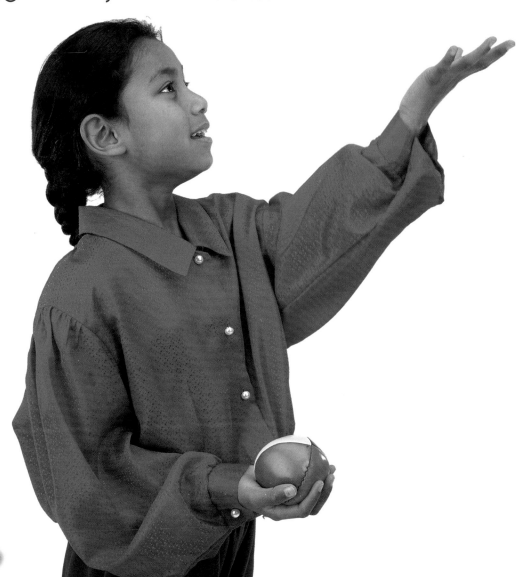

Some jugglers can juggle with any objects they are given.
These men are using special juggling clubs.

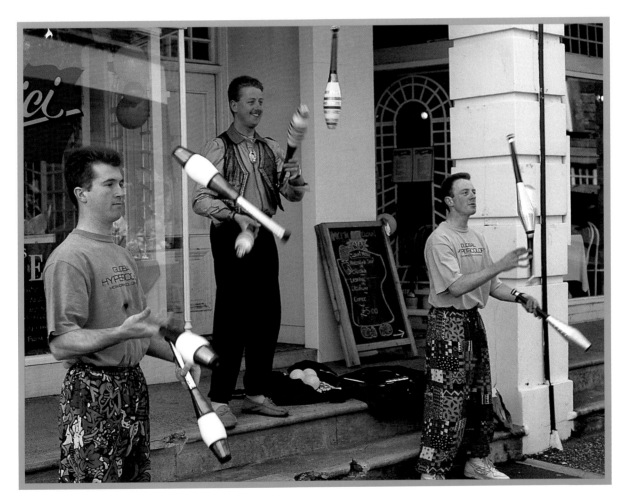

Clown

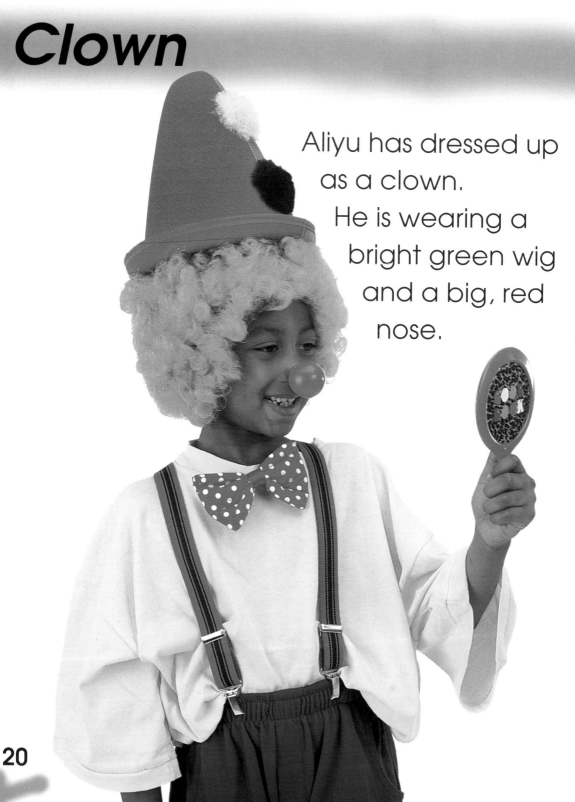

Aliyu has dressed up as a clown.
He is wearing a bright green wig and a big, red nose.

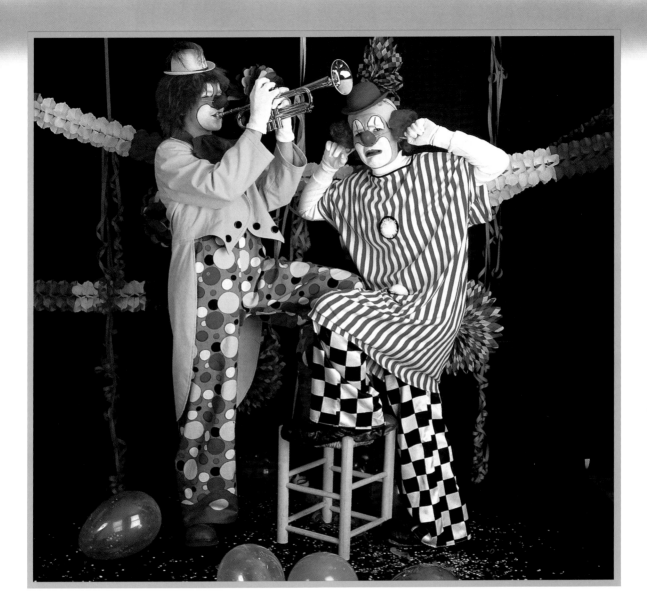

Clowns make people laugh.
They wear funny clothes and do
funny things.

Conductor

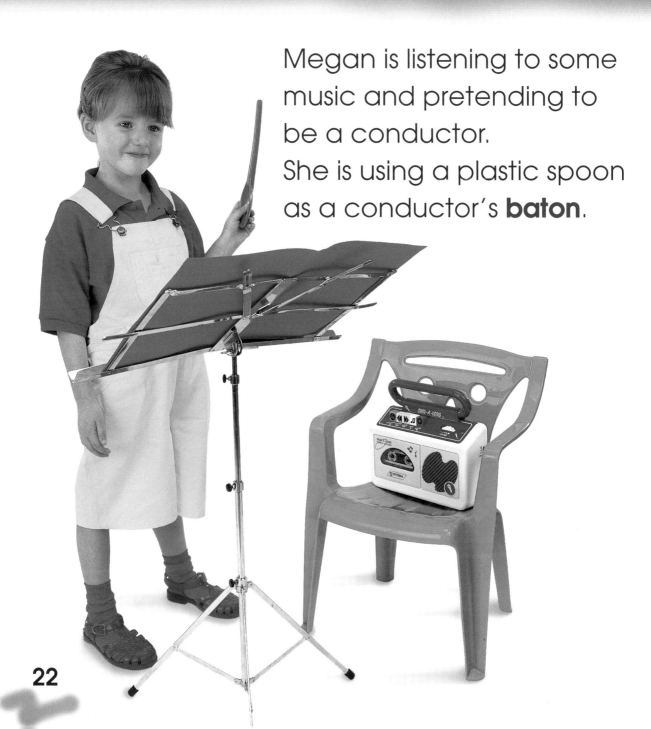

Megan is listening to some music and pretending to be a conductor.
She is using a plastic spoon as a conductor's **baton**.

22

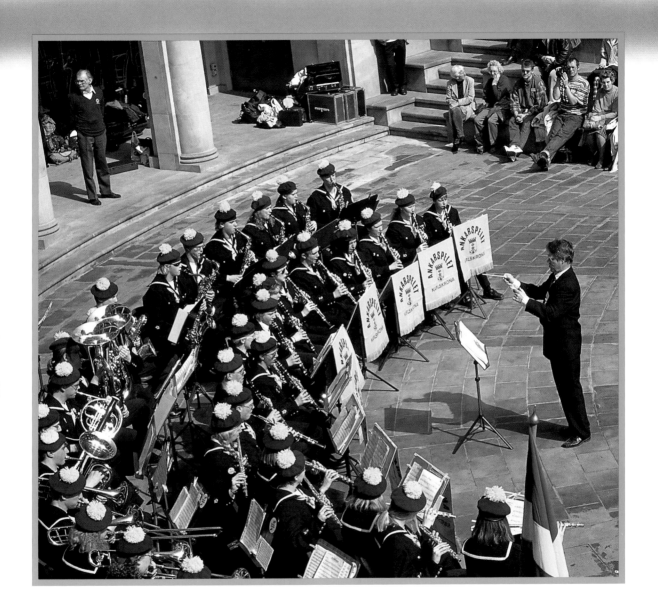

Conductors stand in front of the **orchestra**.
They use a baton to make sure that everyone
plays the music at the same speed.

Glossary

baton   This is a special stick used by a conductor.

hand puppet   A puppet worked by putting your hand inside it is called a hand puppet.

instruments   These are objects that people can use to make music.

marionette   A puppet worked by strings attached to pieces of wood is called a marionette.

old-fashioned   This means something in the style of a long time ago.

orchestra   A group of people who play different musical instruments together are called an orchestra.

tutu   This is a ballet costume with a net skirt.

unicycle   A cycle with only one wheel and a seat is called a unicycle.

Index

More Books to Read

Hudson, Wade. *I'm Gonna Be*. East Orange, NJ: Just US Books, 1992.

Kundstadter, Maria. *Women Working A to Z*. Fort Atkinson, WI: Highsmith Press, 1994.

Scarry, Richard. *What Do People Do All Day?* New York: Random House, 1968.